IBD DIET RECIPES COOKBOOK

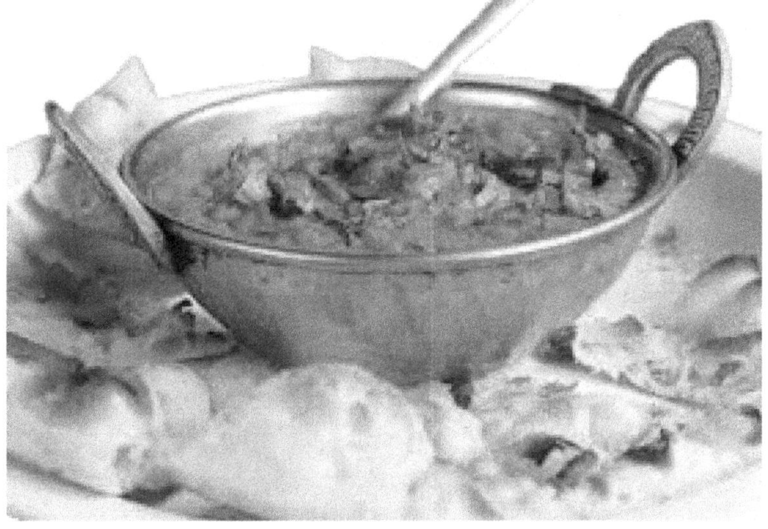

A Comprehensive Guide to Family-Friendly, IBD-Friendly, and Low-FODMAP Recipes for Optimal Gut Health and Wellness

Isabelle Hartley

OTHER BOOKS BY THIS AUTHOR

1. GASTROPARESIS DIET RECIPES COOKBOOK
2. HIGH CALORIES DIET COOKBOOK
3. DIET FOR WOMEN OVER FORTY
4. HASHIMOTO RECIPES COOKBOOK
5. JUICING RECIPES FOR CANCER
6. IVF DIET COOKBOOK FOR BEGINNERS
7. LOW SUGAR DIET GUIDE FOR BEGINNERS
8. RAW FOODS RECIPES COOKBOOK
9. SMOOTHIES RECIPES FOR ANTI-INFLAMMATION
10. MEDITERRANEAN DIET FOR PREGNANT WOMEN

TABLE OF CONTENTS

Introduction

Meet Mark, a resilient individual who embarked on a transformative journey to overcome the challenges posed by Inflammatory Bowel Disease (IBD). Struggling with the debilitating effects of Crohn's disease, Mark decided to explore the potential of dietary changes as a means of managing his condition.

Mark began by consulting with a nutritionist specializing in IBD. Together, they crafted a personalized diet plan focused on anti-inflammatory foods. Mark incorporated nutrient-dense options like leafy greens, lean proteins, and gut-friendly probiotics into his daily meals. He bid farewell to processed foods and embraced whole, unprocessed alternatives, understanding the profound impact of nutrition on his digestive health.

One of the key pillars of Mark's success was adopting a predominantly plant-based diet. He found solace in dishes rich in fiber, such as quinoa, lentils, and a variety of colorful vegetables. These choices not only nourished his body but also supported a balanced gut microbiome, a crucial factor in IBD management.

As weeks passed, Mark experienced a gradual improvement in his symptoms. The frequency and severity of flare-ups diminished, and his energy levels soared. Encouraged by these positive changes, he integrated regular exercise and stress-management techniques into his routine, further enhancing his overall well-being.

Mark's commitment to his newfound lifestyle was unwavering. He educated himself about food triggers and diligently kept a food diary to identify patterns related to his symptoms. This proactive approach empowered him to make informed choices, effectively preventing potential triggers.

Mark's success story serves as an inspiring testament to the transformative power of a well-crafted diet in managing IBD. While his journey wasn't without its challenges, Mark's perseverance, coupled with the right nutritional choices, allowed him not only to manage but significantly improve his quality of life. Today, Mark stands as a beacon of hope for others grappling with IBD, showcasing that a holistic approach to health, including dietary interventions, can pave the way to a brighter, symptom-free future.

CHAPTER 1: IBD DIET

In the intricate tapestry of human health, the gut plays a pivotal role, serving as a hub for digestion, nutrient absorption, and a complex interplay of microorganisms. However, for those navigating the challenging terrain of Inflammatory Bowel Disease (IBD), the delicate balance within this digestive realm is disrupted, giving rise to a spectrum of discomfort, inflammation, and a quest for effective management. Recognizing the profound impact of diet on IBD has prompted a surge of interest and exploration into the realm of tailored nutritional strategies, paving the way for what is commonly known as the IBD diet.

IBD encompasses two primary conditions: Crohn's disease and ulcerative colitis. These disorders manifest as chronic inflammation of the gastrointestinal tract, marked by unpredictable flare-ups and periods of remission. While medical interventions remain a cornerstone in IBD treatment, the importance of diet in alleviating symptoms, managing flare-ups, and promoting overall well-being cannot be overstated.

The journey towards understanding and implementing an IBD-specific diet is a nuanced exploration, weaving through dietary choices, nutrient optimization, and a mindfulness towards individualized triggers. In this comprehensive guide, we embark on a journey to unravel the intricacies of the IBD diet, shedding light on the transformative potential it holds for those seeking to reclaim control over their digestive health.

Recognizing the Role of Nutrition in IBD

At the heart of the IBD diet lies a profound recognition of the symbiotic relationship between nutrition and the gastrointestinal system. While the precise etiology of IBD remains elusive, research indicates that a combination of genetic predisposition, environmental factors, and an aberrant immune response contribute to its onset. Amidst these complex factors, diet emerges as a modifiable element that can influence the course of the disease.

The first step in navigating the IBD diet is acknowledging that there is no one-size-fits-all solution. Each individual's response to dietary interventions can vary, necessitating a personalized approach. It's about deciphering the unique language of one's body, understanding triggers, and crafting a nourishing regimen that aligns with both the nutritional needs and sensitivities of the individual.

Unveiling the IBD Diet Blueprint

The IBD diet blueprint is not a rigid set of rules but a flexible framework, emphasizing nutrient-dense, anti-inflammatory foods while steering clear of potential triggers. Whole, unprocessed foods take center stage, offering a spectrum of vitamins, minerals, and antioxidants essential for overall health. Embracing a predominantly plant-based diet rich in fruits, vegetables, whole grains, and lean proteins forms the cornerstone of this nutritional approach.

Navigating the Nutritional Landscape

A crucial aspect of the IBD diet involves navigating the nutritional landscape with a discerning eye. Certain foods have been identified as potential triggers for IBD symptoms, and individuals are encouraged to keep a food diary to pinpoint specific culprits. Common triggers may include dairy products, spicy foods, high-fiber foods, and certain artificial additives.

In contrast, foods with anti-inflammatory properties become allies in the quest for symptom management. Omega-3 fatty acids, found in fatty fish such as salmon and flaxseeds, showcase potent anti-inflammatory effects. Probiotic-rich foods, including yogurt and fermented options, contribute to a balanced gut microbiome, fostering a supportive environment for digestive health.

While the IBD diet places a spotlight on nutritional choices, its efficacy is amplified when integrated into a broader lifestyle approach. Regular exercise, stress management, and sufficient sleep all contribute to overall well-being and can positively impact IBD symptoms. Understanding the interconnectedness of these lifestyle factors empowers individuals to holistically nurture their health and cultivate resilience in the face of IBD challenges.

In conclusion, the IBD diet represents not just a dietary regimen but a holistic approach to well-being. It is a journey of self-discovery, where individuals learn to listen to their bodies, make informed choices, and adapt to the ever-changing landscape of their health. This comprehensive guide aims to provide insights, practical tips, and inspiration for those navigating the intricate path of the IBD diet. As we delve into the nuances of this transformative journey, may it serve as a beacon of hope and empowerment for those seeking to nourish their bodies, manage their symptoms, and embrace a life of wellness despite the challenges posed by Inflammatory Bowel Disease.

CHAPTER 2: INFLAMMATORY BOWEL DISEASE (IBD

In the intricate landscape of gastrointestinal disorders, Inflammatory Bowel Disease (IBD) stands as a multifaceted challenge, impacting millions of lives worldwide. Characterized by chronic inflammation of the digestive tract, IBD manifests in two primary forms: Crohn's disease and ulcerative colitis. Understanding the causes, symptoms, and distinct characteristics of these conditions is pivotal for effective management and improved quality of life for those grappling with IBD.

Causes of Inflammatory Bowel Disease

While the exact etiology of IBD remains elusive, a complex interplay of genetic, environmental, and immune factors is believed to contribute to its onset. There is a notable genetic predisposition, as individuals with a family history of IBD are at an elevated risk. Specific gene mutations associated with the regulation of the immune system and the gut's ability to tolerate the microbial environment have been identified as potential contributors.

Environmental factors further fuel the intricate dance leading to IBD. Factors such as diet, smoking, and exposure to certain infections or antibiotics may influence disease development. The gut microbiome, a diverse community of microorganisms residing in the digestive tract, also plays a crucial role. Imbalances in this microbial community can trigger an abnormal immune response, sparking inflammation characteristic of IBD.

Symptoms of Inflammatory Bowel Disease

The symptoms of IBD can vary widely, both in type and severity, making diagnosis and management a complex process. Common symptoms include abdominal pain, diarrhea, weight loss, and fatigue. The nature of these symptoms can fluctuate, with periods of active flare-ups interspersed with periods of remission, during which individuals may experience fewer or milder symptoms.

Abdominal pain is a hallmark of IBD, often occurring in the lower right side for individuals with Crohn's disease and throughout the abdomen for those with ulcerative colitis. Diarrhea, sometimes accompanied by blood or mucus, is another prevalent symptom, reflecting the inflammation and damage to the digestive tract.

Weight loss can result from a combination of factors, including decreased appetite, nutrient malabsorption, and the energy expended in battling the chronic inflammation. Fatigue, a pervasive and often underestimated symptom, may arise from the body's continuous efforts to heal and the strain of managing persistent symptoms.

Beyond the digestive symptoms, IBD can manifest in extraintestinal complications, affecting various systems in the body. These may include joint pain, skin rashes, eye inflammation, and liver disorders, underscoring the systemic nature of the disease.

Types of Inflammatory Bowel Disease

Two primary types of IBD, Crohn's disease and ulcerative colitis, share similarities in symptoms but exhibit distinct characteristics in terms of the location and nature of inflammation within the digestive tract.

Crohn's Disease

Crohn's disease is a chronic condition marked by inflammation that can affect any part of the gastrointestinal tract, from the mouth to the anus. This inflammation is often characterized by "skip lesions," meaning segments of healthy tissue can exist between inflamed portions. The layers of the bowel wall may be involved, leading to complications such as strictures, abscesses, and fistulas.

The symptoms of Crohn's disease can vary depending on the specific location and extent of inflammation. Common presentations include abdominal pain, diarrhea, weight loss, and fatigue. Individuals with Crohn's disease may also experience nutritional deficiencies due to impaired absorption in the inflamed portions of the intestine.

Ulcerative Colitis

Ulcerative colitis, on the other hand, is characterized by inflammation predominantly in the colon and rectum. Unlike Crohn's disease, the inflammation in ulcerative colitis is continuous and typically starts in the rectum, extending progressively along the colon. This continuous inflammation may lead to the formation of ulcers on the inner lining of the colon.

The symptoms of ulcerative colitis often include bloody diarrhea, abdominal cramps, and an urgent need to evacuate the bowels. The inflammation in this condition primarily affects the superficial layers of the colon wall. In severe cases, complications such as toxic megacolon, perforation of the colon, or an increased risk of colon cancer may arise.

Diagnostic Challenges and Collaborative Management

Diagnosing IBD involves a combination of clinical evaluation, medical imaging, and laboratory tests. Endoscopic procedures, such as colonoscopy and upper endoscopy, are instrumental in visualizing the extent of inflammation and obtaining tissue samples for a definitive diagnosis.

Management of IBD is a dynamic process that often requires a collaborative effort between healthcare providers, including gastroenterologists, dietitians, and other specialists. Treatment strategies aim to induce and maintain remission, alleviate symptoms, and prevent complications. Medications, including anti-inflammatory drugs, immunosuppressants, and biologics, are commonly prescribed based on the severity and type of IBD.

The role of diet in managing IBD is increasingly recognized, with many individuals finding relief through tailored nutritional approaches. Specific dietary modifications, such as adopting a low-residue or low-FODMAP diet, may be recommended to reduce the frequency and severity of symptoms. It's crucial for individuals to work closely with healthcare professionals to identify triggers, address nutritional deficiencies, and navigate dietary choices that align with their unique needs.

Beyond the physical challenges, IBD can take a toll on mental health. The chronic nature of the disease, unpredictable flare-ups, and the impact on daily life can lead to stress, anxiety, and depression. Recognizing and addressing the emotional aspects of living with IBD is integral to holistic management. Support from healthcare professionals, mental health specialists, and peer communities can provide valuable resources for coping with the emotional impact of the disease.

The landscape of IBD research is dynamic, with ongoing efforts to unravel the complexities of the disease. Advances in genetics, immunology, and microbiome research offer promising insights into potential therapeutic targets. Clinical trials exploring novel medications and interventions contribute to the evolving arsenal of treatment options.

As our understanding of IBD deepens, there is hope for more targeted and personalized approaches to management. The integration of precision medicine, tailored dietary interventions, and advancements in therapeutic options holds the promise of improved outcomes and an enhanced quality of life for individuals navigating the intricate journey of Inflammatory Bowel Disease.

Inflammatory Bowel Disease, with its intricate tapestry of causes, symptoms, and types, underscores the need for a comprehensive and personalized approach to diagnosis and management. The journey of those living with IBD is marked by resilience, adaptation, and a quest for a balanced life despite the challenges. With a collaborative healthcare team, a nuanced understanding of triggers, and advancements in research and therapeutics, individuals can navigate the path forward, striving for remission, improved quality of life, and a hopeful horizon in the evolving landscape of IBD.

CHAPTER 3

Benefits of Adopting the IBD Diet

Embracing the Inflammatory Bowel Disease (IBD) diet offers a myriad of benefits, empowering individuals to proactively manage their symptoms, promote overall well-being, and foster a sense of control over the complex challenges posed by IBD.

Symptom Management: Tailoring one's diet to align with IBD recommendations can lead to a significant reduction in the frequency and severity of symptoms. By avoiding potential triggers and incorporating anti-inflammatory foods, individuals often experience relief from abdominal pain, diarrhea, and fatigue associated with IBD.

Nutritional Support: IBD can impact nutrient absorption and lead to deficiencies. The IBD diet emphasizes nutrient-dense foods, providing essential vitamins, minerals, and antioxidants. This targeted nutritional approach helps address deficiencies and supports overall health, contributing to improved energy levels and vitality.

Gut Microbiome Balance: The IBD diet promotes a healthy balance of the gut microbiome, crucial for digestive health. Probiotic-rich foods and a focus on fiber from fruits and vegetables contribute to a diverse and thriving microbial community, enhancing the gut's ability to maintain equilibrium.

Reduced Inflammation: Chronic inflammation is a hallmark of IBD, contributing to the progression of the disease. The anti-inflammatory nature of the IBD diet, with its emphasis on omega-3 fatty acids, antioxidants, and gut-friendly foods, may help mitigate inflammation, providing relief and potentially slowing the course of the disease.

Improved Quality of Life: Adopting the IBD diet is not just about managing symptoms; it's about reclaiming a sense of normalcy and improving overall quality of life. With a well-balanced nutritional approach, individuals often find they can engage more fully in daily activities, work, and social interactions, fostering a positive mindset.

Complications of Not Adopting the Right Diet

On the flip side, neglecting to adopt the appropriate diet for IBD can lead to a range of complications, exacerbating symptoms and potentially contributing to the progression of the disease.

Increased Symptom Severity: Without dietary modifications, individuals with IBD may experience heightened severity and frequency of symptoms. Persistent abdominal pain, diarrhea, and fatigue can significantly impact daily life, limiting productivity and overall well-being.

Nutritional Deficiencies: IBD often interferes with the absorption of nutrients, leading to deficiencies in essential vitamins and minerals. Neglecting a targeted nutritional approach may exacerbate these deficiencies, contributing to weakness, anemia, and compromised immune function.

Gut Microbiome Imbalance: A diet devoid of gut-friendly foods can contribute to an imbalance in the gut microbiome. This dysbiosis may exacerbate inflammation, weaken the gut barrier, and contribute to the perpetuation of IBD symptoms.

Compromised Immune Response: The immune system plays a central role in IBD, and dietary choices can influence immune function. Without the support of an anti-inflammatory diet, the immune response may become dysregulated, potentially contributing to increased inflammation and disease activity.

Mental Health Impact: Chronic conditions like IBD often have a profound impact on mental health. Failure to adopt a supportive diet can contribute to heightened stress, anxiety, and depression, further compromising the overall well-being of individuals living with IBD.

In summary, the benefits of adopting the IBD diet extend beyond mere symptom management, encompassing a holistic approach to well-being. On the other hand, complications arising from neglecting the right dietary choices underscore the importance of proactive and personalized nutritional strategies in the journey of individuals grappling with Inflammatory Bowel Disease.

Tips for Successful Meal Planning and Preparation in IBD Management

Meal planning and preparation play a crucial role in managing Inflammatory Bowel Disease (IBD), helping individuals navigate dietary choices and minimize potential triggers. Here are essential tips for a successful and supportive approach:

Keep a Food Diary: Track your daily food intake and note any symptoms. This helps identify potential triggers and allows for informed adjustments to your diet. Record not only the types of food but also portion sizes and meal timings.

Focus on Variety: Aim for a diverse and balanced diet that includes a range of fruits, vegetables, whole grains, lean proteins, and healthy fats. Variety ensures you receive a broad spectrum of nutrients, supporting overall health and well-being.

Small, Frequent Meals: Opt for smaller, more frequent meals rather than large, infrequent ones. This approach can be gentler on the digestive system, helping to manage symptoms such as bloating and discomfort.

Hydrate Adequately: Proper hydration is crucial for digestive health. Drink plenty of water throughout the day to maintain hydration and support the optimal functioning of the digestive tract.

Mindful Eating Practices: Cultivate mindful eating habits by savoring each bite, chewing thoroughly, and paying attention to hunger and fullness cues. This can enhance digestion and reduce the likelihood of overeating.

Experiment with Cooking Techniques: Explore different cooking methods, such as steaming, baking, or grilling, to find what works best for you. Some individuals with IBD find that certain cooking techniques are gentler on the digestive system.

Prep Ahead for Convenience: Plan and prep meals in advance to streamline your eating routine. Batch cooking on days when you feel well can provide ready-to-eat options during flare-ups, reducing the stress of meal preparation.

Consider Specific Diets: Explore diets that align with IBD management, such as low-residue or low-FODMAP diets. These approaches can help reduce the frequency and severity of symptoms by limiting certain types of foods that may be triggers.

Communication with Healthcare Providers: Maintain open communication with your healthcare team, including gastroenterologists and dietitians. Share your meal plans and any changes in symptoms, allowing for adjustments and personalized guidance.

Be Flexible and Listen to Your Body: Recognize that dietary needs may evolve. Be flexible with your meal plans and listen to your body's signals. If a particular food consistently triggers symptoms, consider adjusting your diet accordingly.

By incorporating these tips into your meal planning and preparation routine, you can empower yourself to navigate the complexities of IBD with greater ease. Remember that individual responses to foods vary, so it's essential to tailor these strategies to your unique needs and preferences.

Conclusion

In the intricate journey of managing Inflammatory Bowel Disease (IBD), the role of a carefully crafted diet emerges as a powerful ally. From understanding the causes and symptoms to exploring the nuances of the IBD diet, individuals embark on a transformative path toward enhanced well-being and improved quality of life.

The IBD diet, with its focus on anti-inflammatory, nutrient-dense foods and personalized approaches, offers a beacon of hope for those navigating the challenges of Crohn's disease and ulcerative colitis. Through the adoption of mindful eating practices, small, frequent meals, and a variety of nourishing options, individuals can actively manage symptoms, support gut health, and foster resilience in the face of this complex condition.

Successful meal planning and preparation become integral components of the IBD journey, providing individuals with practical tools to navigate dietary choices, identify triggers, and maintain consistency even during flare-ups. Keeping a food diary, experimenting with cooking techniques, and staying hydrated contribute to a holistic approach to managing IBD symptoms.

As we conclude this exploration, it's crucial to recognize the profound impact that the IBD diet can have on overall well-being. Beyond the physical benefits, adopting and adapting to this diet is an empowering step toward reclaiming control over one's life. It's a declaration of resilience, a commitment to self-care, and a recognition that despite the challenges, there exists a path to a more vibrant and fulfilling life.

So, dear reader, consider this not just as a dietary regimen but as a transformative journey—one that holds the potential to reshape your relationship with food, empower your body, and nurture your spirit. Embrace the IBD diet not as a restriction but as a pathway to healing, a canvas on which you can paint a portrait of wellness. With each mindful bite, each well-prepared meal, you are taking steps toward a healthier, more vibrant future. You have the strength to navigate this journey, and the IBD diet is a valuable tool in your arsenal. Let it be a source of inspiration, motivation, and a testament to your resilience. Your journey toward well-being is a unique narrative, and the IBD diet is here to support you every step of the way.

Contact Us

Dear Reader,

If you have any questions, need further clarification, or require assistance with any aspect of the book, please do not hesitate to reach out to me. I am more than happy to provide additional insights, address your queries, or simply engage in a meaningful discussion.

Feel free to contact me at: IsabelleHartleyBooks@gmail.com. Your feedback and inquiries are always welcome.

FREE 30 DAY MEAL PLANNER

DAILY MEAL PLANNER

Day:

BREAKFAST

LUNCH

DINNER

INGREDIENTS NEEDED

DAILY MEAL PLANNER

Day: ....

BREAKFAST

LUNCH

DINNER

INGREDIENTS NEEDED

- [ ]
- [ ]
- [ ]
- [ ]

DAILY MEAL PLANNER

Day: ....

BREAKFAST

LUNCH

DINNER

INGREDIENTS NEEDED

DAILY MEAL PLANNER

Day: ....

BREAKFAST

____

____

LUNCH

____

____

DINNER

____

____

INGREDIENTS NEEDED

☐ _______________________________________

☐ _______________________________________

☐ _______________________________________

☐ _______________________________________

DAILY MEAL PLANNER

Day:

BREAKFAST

LUNCH

DINNER

INGREDIENTS NEEDED

DAILY MEAL PLANNER

Day: ....

BREAKFAST

LUNCH

DINNER

INGREDIENTS NEEDED

- [ ]
- [ ]
- [ ]
- [ ]

DAILY MEAL PLANNER

Day: ....

BREAKFAST

LUNCH

DINNER

INGREDIENTS NEEDED

- [ ]
- [ ]
- [ ]
- [ ]

DAILY MEAL PLANNER

Day:

BREAKFAST

LUNCH

DINNER

INGREDIENTS NEEDED

- [ ]
- [ ]
- [ ]
- [ ]

DAILY MEAL PLANNER

Day: ....

BREAKFAST

LUNCH

DINNER

INGREDIENTS NEEDED

- [ ]
- [ ]
- [ ]
- [ ]

DAILY MEAL PLANNER

Day: ....

BREAKFAST

LUNCH

DINNER

INGREDIENTS NEEDED

DAILY MEAL PLANNER

Day: ....

BREAKFAST

LUNCH

DINNER

INGREDIENTS NEEDED

- [ ]
- [ ]
- [ ]
- [ ]

DAILY MEAL PLANNER

Day: ....

BREAKFAST

LUNCH

DINNER

INGREDIENTS NEEDED

DAILY MEAL PLANNER

Day: ....

BREAKFAST

____

____

LUNCH

____

____

DINNER

____

____

INGREDIENTS NEEDED

☐ ____

☐ ____

☐ ____

☐ ____

DAILY MEAL PLANNER

Day: ....

BREAKFAST

LUNCH

DINNER

INGREDIENTS NEEDED

- [ ]
- [ ]
- [ ]
- [ ]

DAILY MEAL PLANNER

Day:

BREAKFAST

LUNCH

DINNER

INGREDIENTS NEEDED

DAILY MEAL PLANNER

Day:

BREAKFAST

LUNCH

DINNER

INGREDIENTS NEEDED

DAILY MEAL PLANNER

Day: ....

BREAKFAST

LUNCH

DINNER

INGREDIENTS NEEDED

- [ ]
- [ ]
- [ ]
- [ ]

DAILY MEAL PLANNER

Day: ....

BREAKFAST

LUNCH

DINNER

INGREDIENTS NEEDED

DAILY MEAL PLANNER

Day:

BREAKFAST

LUNCH

DINNER

INGREDIENTS NEEDED

DAILY MEAL PLANNER

Day: ....

BREAKFAST

LUNCH

DINNER

INGREDIENTS NEEDED

☐
☐
☐
☐

DAILY MEAL PLANNER

Day: ....

BREAKFAST

____

____

LUNCH

____

____

DINNER

____

____

INGREDIENTS NEEDED

☐ _______________________________________

☐ _______________________________________

☐ _______________________________________

☐ _______________________________________

DAILY MEAL PLANNER

Day:

BREAKFAST

LUNCH

DINNER

INGREDIENTS NEEDED

DAILY MEAL PLANNER

Day:

BREAKFAST

LUNCH

DINNER

INGREDIENTS NEEDED

DAILY MEAL PLANNER

Day:

BREAKFAST

LUNCH

DINNER

INGREDIENTS NEEDED

DAILY MEAL PLANNER

Day:

BREAKFAST

LUNCH

DINNER

INGREDIENTS NEEDED

DAILY MEAL PLANNER

Day:

BREAKFAST

LUNCH

DINNER

INGREDIENTS NEEDED

DAILY MEAL PLANNER

Day: ....

BREAKFAST

____

____

LUNCH

____

____

DINNER

____

____

INGREDIENTS NEEDED

☐ ____

☐ ____

☐ ____

☐ ____

DAILY MEAL PLANNER

Day:

BREAKFAST

LUNCH

DINNER

INGREDIENTS NEEDED

DAILY MEAL PLANNER

Day: ....

BREAKFAST

____

____

LUNCH

____

____

DINNER

____

____

INGREDIENTS NEEDED

☐ _______________________________

☐ _______________________________

☐ _______________________________

☐ _______________________________

DAILY MEAL PLANNER

Day: ....

BREAKFAST

____

____

LUNCH

____

____

DINNER

____

____

INGREDIENTS NEEDED

☐ _______________________________

☐ _______________________________

☐ _______________________________

☐ _______________________________

www.ingramcontent.com/pod-product-compliance
Lightning Source LLC
Chambersburg PA
CBHW071103260726
48661CB00006B/2437